Table of Contents

2018 Update Road to Recovery from Parkinsons Disease

2018 Update Road to Recovery from Parkinsons Disease

Important Disclaimer

I am not a medical doctor. I am a PhD type researcher. Please do not take anything I might say or write as medical advice. I am not qualified to diagnose or treat disease. My perspective is based purely on a research perspective.

Please. Consult with your doctor and/or health care provider before deciding whether to take action on any of the new therapies reviewed in this 2018 update. The therapies I review here really are all recent discoveries or inventions. This means there is little systematic evidence (in most cases) for many of the therapies reviewed here. Please do your own due diligence.

Robert Rodgers PhD
Parkinsons Recovery
https://www.parkinsonsrecovery.com

Truth of Recovery Really is Simple

My research agenda for the past decade and a half has been to identify natural therapies that offer the promise of helping people reverse the symptoms associated with a diagnosis of Parkinson's disease. In part, this initiative has involved airing 250 interviews with health care professionals, doctors and therapists who have offered remarkable suggestions for what has been helping people recover. All of these radio show interviews are available as replays for free. Links to the more recent interviews are provided in this update.

- What is the bottom line of this extensive research?

- What is the truth of recovery?

- Is it complicated?

Most people think it must be. Or, is it simple? I have concluded the key to a successful recovery is

actually very simple indeed. I did not believe this
a decade ago.

Seventy of the 250 interviews I have hosted on my
radio program have been with guests diagnosed
with Parkinson's disease who discovered one way
or another to find relief from their symptoms. The
surprise to me as a researcher has been the vastly
different paths individuals have taken to engage a
successful journey down the road to recovery.
Each story is unique.

What do these remarkable pioneers of recovery
have in common? They report radically different
specifics of their individual recovery programs.
Listen to some of the replays of the interviews and
you will begin to appreciate how each person
discovered their own best course of therapies that
helped them heal.

Despite the differences, I recently asked the
question: What do these pioneers of recovery
have in common? The answer will shock you.
Using a vast variety of approaches and therapies

they all found ways to infuse their body with the basics of life – light, water, oxygen and grounding.

Without the light of the sun there would be no life.

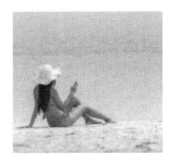

Without oxygen from the air we breathe there would be no life

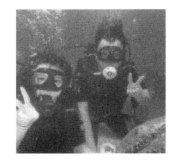

Without water to drink, there would be no life.

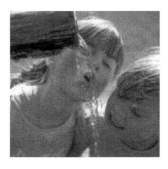

Without grounding to mother earth, we are truly lost.

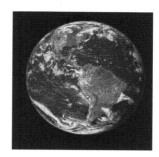

The authentic answer to recovery turns out to be profoundly simple. A body that is struggling with neurological difficulties is not receiving sufficient light, water, oxygen, grounding (or all four). Fortunately there have been a number of exciting developments that enable the rich and safe infusion of light and oxygen into the cells of the body as well as homeopathic remedies that have been designed to hydrate cells.

As I now see it, success with a recovery program depends on giving your body what it needs to thrive – light, water, oxygen and grounding. It really is that simple folks.

Light Therapy

Researchers have recently found evidence that light therapy is a promising therapy for persons experiencing the symptoms of Parkinson's disease. The retina is believed to play a pivotal role in the nigrostriatal dopamine system. Light (obviously) passes through the eyes and shines on the retina which happens to be a close neighbor of the substantia nigra, the organ positioned in the middle of the brain. I have drawn the logical conclusion is that - Duh - light should of course make a difference!

A study by researchers at the Bronowski Clinic in Australia conducted a longitudinal study of 129 patients diagnosed with Parkinson's disease. Subjects who were classified as compliant - meaning they used light therapy regularly - exhibited significant improvement over subjects that were partially compliant or non-compliant.

An encouraging observation of the compliant subjects was that the drug burden was less with fewer side effects. These findings suggest that light therapy shows promise as an option to address symptoms of Parkinson's and a therapy which might potentially reduce the role of medications to suppress symptoms.

What is Photobiomodulation?

Neurons are cells that contain mitochondria. Photobiomodulation energizes neuronal mitochondria, triggering a cascade of beneficial cellular functions. Potential benefits are neuroprotective effects, self-repair mechanisms and enhanced functionality.

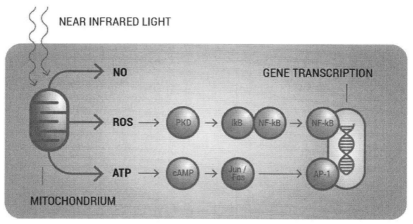

CELLULAR MECHANISMS

Reference: "Basic Photomedicine", Ying-Ying Huang, Pawel Mroz, and Michael R. Hamblin, Harvard Medical School.

Visible red and near infrared light energy stimulates cells to generate more energy facilitating self-repair. The healing takes place within the mitochondria through an enzyme called cytochrome c oxidase. This enzyme accepts and converts the light (or photonic) energy into cellular energy (ATP) and other gene transcription factors leading to cellular repair and regeneration.

Research on Light Therapy from MIT

The following video previews recent research at MIT that explains why light therapy offers a promising opportunity to reverse dementia associated with a diagnosis of Alzheimer's disease.

https://www.youtube.com/watch?v=O_p4QWkE2Ls

Intranasal photobiomodulation is the most efficient method for light energy to reach the brain. Different from electrical and magnetic stimulation, photobiomodulation uses light energy (or photons) of specific wave lengths and power density to simulate cellular function. One such invention was developed by Vielight located in Toronto Canada.

https://www.youtube.com/watch?v=jroi70LXpLI

Vielight Photobiomodulation Gamma Device
Recent research developments have led me to conclude that the future of medicine in part rests with innovative therapies that utilize light to bring the body back into balance and harmony. A recent invention, the Vielight photobiomodulation Gamma Device, is one such development that redirects our understanding of how symptoms can be addressed successfully.

I interviewed the inventor of this new light therapy device on Parkinsons Recovery Radio October of 2017. Click below to hear my interview with Lew Lim:

Lew Lim PhD Answers Questions on Parkinsons Recovery Radio

What has been the experience of persons with Parkinson's symptoms who have been using the Vielight Gamma Device?

So far, sixty-one (61) persons who listened to my interview on the Vielight device purchased the unit using the 10% coupon code (**healing4me**) Dr. Lim provided to my listeners. Those who acquired the device were invited to return the device to the company after using it for six months if it did not offer relief from their symptoms and receive an 80% refund of the purchase price.

The company reported to me that five of the Neuro Gamma unites have been returned thus far. One crude estimate of effectiveness is that approximately 90% of users are satisfied it helps address some symptoms.

I have also heard from a member of my audience who lives in Ecuador who is connected with a community of persons with Parkinson's symptoms. He reports that virtually all users experienced welcome relief from some symptoms. For some, the most pronounced results were seen in the initial four (4) months or so after which the improvements tended to level off.

Anecdotal Reports about the Vielight Photobiomodulation Neuro Device as a Treatment for Parkinson's Symptoms

There is currently no systematic published research on the use of the Vielight Gamma Photobiomodulation device as a therapy to specifically address Parkinson's symptoms. As a new invention, this is certainly not surprising. I have heard informal feedback from users who are members of the Parkinsons Recovery audience that the therapy has resulted in relief of some symptoms and report below my summary observations:

1. One common report from users is that the therapy does not show quick results. You apparently have to apply the therapy over a period of several weeks to a month or longer to celebrate a positive shift in symptoms.

2. I have heard several specific reports on tremors that were calmed.

3. It is unclear at this point to what degree the therapy will address balance issues, but I have heard it seems to offer help with gait challenges.

4. Evidence does suggest that this therapy can potentially help with dementia.

5. One user reported a definite return of smell, but the jury was out on the effect on tremors and other symptoms.

6. The wife of one 85 year old man with advanced Parkinson's symptoms reported that after 6 weeks of using the Vielight Neuro device there were no major improvements but several minor ones of some consequence: Her husband reports being more alert, sleeping better, his cough is less, he has been inspired lately to use his automatic peddler and his hallucinations have dwindled. She reports it has been an answer for a better quality of life for both of them and promises to keep me updated.

2018 Update Road to Recovery from Parkinsons Disease

Of course, it is difficult for people diagnosed with Parkinson's to attribute an improvement in symptoms directly to their photobiomodulation therapy when they are getting other therapies at the same time. Reports above are a general summary of the informal feedback I have received in emails and phone conversations. One person told me it did not offer them the relief they had expected and returned the unit.

Like virtually all natural therapies I have documented over the past 14 years, the Vielight Neuro Gamma device will not help everyone. Odds do appear to be in your favor if you decide to try it out. I predict Dr. Lim's new invention promises to set health care in new and exciting directions and has the potential to offer far reaching benefits to many persons (but not all!) who currently experience Parkinson's symptoms.

Dr. Lew Lim is an engineer and a Doctor of Natural Medicine with additional diplomas in Medical Neuroscience and Business and Accountancy. He obtained his degrees and diplomas from the University of California at Berkeley, University of

Sheffield, Duke University, Quantum University and The Chartered Institute of Management Accountants, UK.

https://www.youtube.com/watch?v=hXChKGvMHw0

Photobiomodulation Research

A 2017 study examined the effects of photobiomodulation (PBM), a light therapy that uses red or near-infrared light to heal and protect tissues, in five older adults with dementia, one of the symptoms of Parkinson's.

After 12 weeks of treatment subjects showed significant improvements on the Cognitive Alzheimer's Disease Assessment Scale. With only five subjects, the effect sizes had to be huge for significance to be shown. This suggests that symptoms most likely to be helped are memory issues, brain fog and occasional confusion.

Caregivers who kept daily journals tracking experiences of the five research subjects reported participants had:

2018 Update Road to Recovery from Parkinsons Disease

- Better sleep
- Fewer angry outbursts
- Decreased anxiety

Did Positive Results for Subjects Continue After Treatment was Suspended?

No. Precipitous declines were observed during the follow-up 4 week no-treatment period. Results suggest treatments need to continue for results to be sustained.

Saltmarche et al.(2017) **Photomed Laser Surg**. 2017 Aug;35(8)

About the Vielight Photobiomodulation Device

The company, Vielight, has generously offered followers of Parkinsons Recovery a 10% discount off orders of the the Vielight Neuro Gamma device which retails for $1749. Enter the coupon code **healing4me** on the shopping cart on the Vielight website. The website is:
https://www.vielight.com

Vielight Six Month Warranty

Vielight is so confident in its new product that you get six (6) months to try out their newly invented photobiomodulation therapy. If for any reason you are not satisfied, you can return it for a 80%

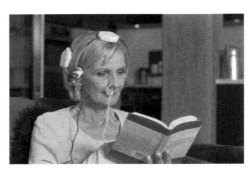

refund. I have never heard of a company that is so confident in their product that such a generous warranty can be extended. They obviously have high confidence in their new invention. While there is scant evidence about its effectiveness for people who experience symptoms of Parkinson's disease, the opportunity to try it out for minimal risk is currently available.

Act Now or Wait for More Evidence?

If you prefer to wait for clear and convincing evidence that this or any light therapy will help with symptoms of Parkinson's disease, be on the lookout for research findings that will be completed and released 5-10 years from now. The instigation of studies takes years and of course costs many millions of dollars.

I would personally prefer to see many people with the symptoms start getting photobiomodulation therapy now. Early users are giving us rich indications about its usefulness as a treatment for Parkinson's symptoms. I do not hesitate to suggest this as a treatment option to take seriously.

Are medicines and/or supplements no longer working for you? If the answer is yes to this question, what treatment options remain? There is, of course, Deep Brain Stimulation available as an option, but I am well aware many of you prefer not to pursue this treatment option. It is my hope and prayer that photobiomodulation therapy will become a natural option that supports the therapeutic effect of medicines and supplements such that the dosage does not have to be increased or even can be reduced under close supervision of your doctor.

2018 Update Road to Recovery from Parkinsons Disease

I do recommend that you consider this therapy so we can discover together whether my prediction of success is right or wrong. Keep in mind that while the device is relatively expensive - $1749 - you:

1. Can claim a 10% discount if you use the Parkinsons Recovery discount code of **healing4me**.
2. Get 6 months of use to see if it offers symptomatic relief or not.
3. Risk is reduced 80% since you can return the device within the 6 month period after purchase for an 80% refund of the purchase price.
4. Everyone in the family can use the therapy.

The Vielight company obviously has confidence in their product which is a very encouraging sign. I have never heard of any company that offered a 6 month warranty. You can purchase the **Gamma Vielight device** from the Vielight website:

www.vielight.com

Be sure to enter the coupon code healing4me on the Vielight shopping cart to claim your Parkinsons Recovery 10% discount. Please also email me your experience with using it after a month (or longer) of use.

Vielight Photobiomodulation Device Instructional Manual Video

https://www.youtube.com/watch?v=BxQSwjnC-E4&t=2s

I hope many of you will try this therapy out and let me know the result. It is not a permanent "fix" to be sure, but neither is medicine. I am attracted to this option because it is noninvasive and inexpensive over the long term when you consider it can be used for a lifetime and by all members of the household.

Will Photobiomodulation Therapy Interfere with My Daily Life?

No. You are welcome to receive the therapy while working, reading or doing anything really. Dr. Lim, the inventor, recommends that people with more serious health issues such as Alzheimer's might be advised to do the therapy at night while going to sleep. The treatment duration lasts only 20 minutes.

2018 Update Road to Recovery from Parkinsons Disease

High Dose Thiamine

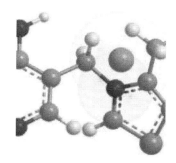

High-Dose Thiamine is promoted by Italian neurologist Antonio Constantini MD but is little known as a therapy in the United States. He has been prescribing High Dose Thiamine as a treatment for his Parkinson's patients with good success. Visit the link below to hear the replay of my interview on Parkinsons Recovery Radio on May 23, 2018 with Dr. Constantini.

<u>Dr. Constantini Discusses High Dose Thiamine as a Therapy for Parkinson's</u>

What follows is a summary of my interview with Dr. Constantini.

What Results have Your Parkinson's Patients Experienced?

It depends in part on whether the person has recently experienced symptoms of Parkinson's or has had them for several years. For the newly diagnosed taking high dose thiamine (whether by oral tablet or injection) reduces motor symptoms on average by 50% to 70%. In selected cases a patient can celebrate experiencing no symptoms. Improvements in motor symptoms are common.

For patients who have experienced symptoms for a long period of time, Dr.Costantini prescribes L-dopa and other more traditional medications. Such patients are also reported to experience symptom relief but results are generally not as dramatic.

How "High" Does the Thiamine Dosage Need to Be?

The recommended dosage varies considerably from patient to patient and is determined only after a medical checkup. Many factors influence the dosage that is prescribed. Possibilities range from 1 gram up to 4 grams a day of Vitamin B1 which is much more than the dose normally recommended.

For some patients requiring the higher doses, Dr. Costantini may administer B1 injections of 100 milligrams twice a week for a total intake of 200 milligrams each week of treatment.

Why Do You Prescribe High Dose Thiamine for Your Parkinson's Patients?

When there is a deficiency of thiamine, the result is a dysfunction in metabolism. For persons experiencing Parkinson's symptoms, Dr. Costantini hypothesized there is a deficiency in the update of thiamine to the brain cells that produce dopamine.

How Quickly Do Parkinson's Patients Begin to Experience Relief from Symptoms?

If they are taking Thiamine in tablet or powder form, it typically takes 2-3 days to experience symptomatic improvement. When shots or injections are administered the improvement can typically be experienced in 30-45 minutes.

Once a patient begins taking high dose thiamine Dr. Costantini reports that they typically must continue taking it to receive continued benefits. It is possible to take short breaks without incurring troublesome setbacks.

What Conditions Other the Parkinson's Is High Dose Thiamine Therapy Useful?

Dr. Costantini reports that high dose thiamine is also useful for chronic fatigue, fibromyalgia, cluster headaches, migraines and Huntington's disease.

I recently Checked My B1 Levels and They are Within Normal Limits

You might well be thinking – OK. I will have my doctor check my thiamine levels (vitamin B1). Maybe my levels are too low. Or, you already know that your levels are within normal limits. End of story for you? Dr. Constantini says no.

In the initial stages of his investigations Dr. Constantini did check thiamine levels in his original patients. He found them to be within normal limits. Wait a minute, eh? If the thiamine levels were within normal limits, why should taking a mega dose of thiamine make a difference? What follows is my explanation of what explains his revelation.

The problem has nothing to do with the actual quantity of B1 vitamin (or any of the series of B vitamins). Rather, the body is not converting the B vitamins that are present in "normal quantities" to the enzymes that are essential for the body function well. In more formal terms, this is known as a breakdown in the methylation cycle.

Breakdown in the Methylation Cycle

Persons diagnosed with Parkinson's disease are more likely to have a breakdown in their methylation cycle. I learned this from conducting a series of interviews with BioAcoustic Pioneer Sharry Edwards who has run a series of bioacoustic diagnostics for persons diagnosed with Parkinson's.

Sharry has identified a surprising number of factors that cause neurological imbalances. One that jumps to the top of the list is a breakdown in the methylation cycle. In simple terms, a person has a sufficient quantity of the B vitamins such as B1, but their body is not converting the B vitamins (and B1 in particular) to the enzymes that are essential for body to function normally.

Once the B vitamins (B1, B2, B3, B6, B9, B12) have been thoroughly processed by the methylation cycle, the body uses various methyl-groups to make healthy cells which result in the production of neurotransmitters such as – you guessed it – dopamine. A fully functioning cycle makes it possible to remove toxins in the liver and elsewhere in addition to fighting infections successfully. In other words, B vitamins play an indirect but essential role in promoting healthy neurons.

Taking a normal dose of B1 and other B vitamins may well not result in the critical conversion to the enzymes that are essential for the body to function. The body has to be loaded with excessive quantities of B1 to override the short circuit in the methylation cycle. The important question turns on the question – what causes the methylation cycle to bomb out?

Why does the Methylation Cycle Short Circuit?

The answer is quite simple: excessive and unrelenting stress. Anyone who experiences Parkinson's symptoms knows that stress has a direct and immediate impact on making symptoms worse. When stressed to the hilt, there is a heavy demand on the methylation cycle. This is why the cycle requires greater quantities of B vitamins to convert the vitamins to enzymes. .

When the methylation cycle is not functioning, you will be fatigued, depressed, irritable, anxious, susceptible to infections and confused. The reason why the detox therapies have limited success can be often explained by a dysfunctional methylation cycle.

To summarize: The methylation cycle affects:

- Neurotransmitter levels. This is why so many individuals diagnosed with Parkinson's have persistent anxiety and a deep depression that never seems to lift.

- The immune function. This is why so many persons with Parkinson's symptoms get some relief from taking Low Dose Naltrexone which tricks the immune system into becoming stronger.
- Detoxification. This is why so many individuals have pursued one detox regime after another with limited success. The problem does not reside with the detox protocols per se, but a breakdown in the methylation cycle.
- Production of Glutathione (which is a major antioxidant and protector of your cells). This is why so many persons diagnosed with Parkinson's are known to have dangerously low levels of glutathione.

Since the methylation cycle has been compromised or worse, side lined, a therapy that appears to offer promise (in light of Dr. Costantini's research) is to take mega doses of vitamin B1 (thiamine) to support the function of the methylation cycle. "Normal levels" are insufficient to activate the cycle. Most of the unused reside from B1 is eliminated rather than used to creates enzymes.

Food Sources of Thiamine

After announcing my interview with Antonio Costantini MD I received the following email from Aunt Bean regarding natural food sources of Thiamine (or Vitamin B1) as a therapy for Parkinson's. As you will see below Aunt Bean has found eating foods that contain high concentrations of thiamine reduce her requirements for the fava bean natural dopamine supplement she takes. (She makes her own fava bean tincture).

Aunt Bean refers to her natural l-dopa tincture in her correspondence to me that is copied below. The natural dopamine supplement Aunt Bean is referring to in her email is the tincture she invented using fava beans. Visit the fava bean Parkinsons Recovery website to learn all about Aunt Bean's fava bean tincture and her other natural food research discoveries for Parkinson's.

www.favabeans.parkinsonsrecovery.com

What follows is Aunt Bean's Email.

Yes on thiamine Robert. Since I have been eating nuts for a year and 2 months I have reduced my natural l-dopa tincture from 5 a day to usually one time a day.

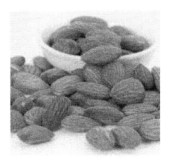

Mandolin playing and strength are much better also. I eat 1 brazil nut, 4 walnut halves, 4 almonds,

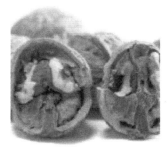

2 bitter apricot kernels, handful of cashews and handful of pistachios a day.

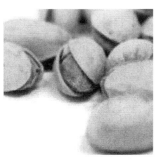

Thumbs up☺.Aunt Bean

2018 Update Road to Recovery from Parkinsons Disease

Pulsed Electromagnetic Field Therapy

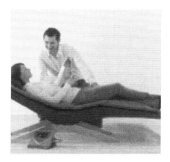

Click on the link below to hear a fascinating radio show interview with Natural Pharmacist Ross Pelton PhD and David Sage who discuss the impressive research documenting the effects of BEMER, an innovative Pulsed Electromagnetic Field Therapy (PEMF) therapy. If your recovery program is stuck in the mud at the present moment, I encourage you to listen to the replay of this informative interview.

http://www.blogtalkradio.com/parkinsons-recovery/2018/02/19/pulsed-electromagnetic-field-therapy

FDA Approval of PEMF Therapy
Below are listed the years when United States FDA has approved specific uses for PEMF Therapy

- 1979 – Non-union fractures
- 1998 – Urinary Incontinence and Muscle Stimulation

- 2004 – Cervical Fusion Patients At High-Risk of Non-Fusion

- 2006 – Depression and Anxiety

- 2011 – Brain Cancer

- 2015 – FDA Upgrade PEMF Classification from Class 3 to Class 2

  In summary, pulsed electromagnetic therapy has been approved by the FDA to promote the healing of various conditions. Electromagnets are used in brain and muscle research to generate currents strong enough to fire nerves that trigger sensations and flex muscles. To date, there have been many research studies and clinical trials on pulsed electro-magnetic field therapy.

Brief PEMF History

PEMF history begins with Nikola Tesla who was the first modern individual recognized for manipulating electromagnetic fields for health purposes. His methods and patents in the early 1900s for the Tesla coil were also used for electromagnetic medical devices.

Five hundred years ago, Paracelsus, a Swiss physician and alchemist, wondered if diseases could be manipulated by magnets using lodestones as the best magnets available then. Natural lodestones have very weak charges. Few people paid much attention to his ideas until the discovery of carbon-steel magnets in the 1700's. During the 1800's discoveries relating electricity to magnetism were made by the early pioneers of our modern technical world including Gauss, Weber, Faraday and Maxwell among others.

The Earth's magnetic field is not fixed in position or strength. It has weakened on the average by about 6 percent over the past 100 years and 30% over the past 1000 years. Some researchers hypothesize that since humans evolved in a magnetic field, it is necessary for proper health. A falling magnetic field puts us at risk. Magnetic therapy helps make up the deficit.

One of the benefits of PEMF is to re-establish healthy cellular membrane potential. This happens when more nutrients are delivered to the cells and when more waste is removed. When the passage ways (the tiny capillaries) which deliver nutrients to the cells and remove waste are restricted and road blocked, membrane potential is seriously compromised.

All About the BEMER Pulsed Electromagnetic Field Therapy

The BEMER is an advanced form of PEMF which is designed to improve circulation thereby supporting the body's natural self-regulating processes. Blood is the body's universal means of transport. Oxygen, nutrients, chemical messengers (e.g., hormones) and immune cells are all transported through our blood. When our body's cells, tissues and organs are adequately nourished and metabolic waste products are removed, our bodies become healthy and function properly. The optimal regulation of circulation is a prerequisite for ensuring good levels of health and fitness.

Veins and arteries enable blood to pass through the tissues of our body. These passageways however constitute only a fourth of the transportation system used to deliver nutrients to the cells and remove waste. Most of the delivery system consists of micro vessels

Research on PEMF reports a series of positive outcomes including modulation of inflammation, reduction of bodily discomforts, promotion of tissue repair and regeneration, improvement of cardiac function, reduction of fatigue, acceleration of recovery from accidents and support of waste removal. These positive outcomes might clearly have a positive benefit for persons currently experiencing neurological challenges.

The BEMER is a patented, FDA-approved device which utilizes Pulsed Electromagnetic Field Therapy. BEMER stands for Bio-Electro-Magnetic-Energy-Regulation.

About the BEMER PRO Kit

The BEMER Pro kit consists of a pad that you lie on or sit on. The electro-magnetic frequencies cause an increase in micro-capillary blood flow. This results in increased delivery of oxygen & nutrients to all cells and improves removal of cellular waste.

The link below takes you to a short video that shows dramatic increase in micro-capillary blood flow after just one 8-minute BEMER session.

https://www.youtube.com/watch?v=0h6_N_HLkgo

Here is a link to a 5-minute video that gives an easy to understand explanation of the BEMER technology.

https://www.youtube.com/watch?v=d9p2-iGMDOo

The suggested protocol for BEMER therapy is just two 8-minute sessions daily. The entire body benefits from increased oxygenation and improved detoxification. This explains why BEMER's ability to enhance micro-capillary circulation helps people with many kinds of health issues. In addition to reducing stiffness, soreness & inflammation, other BEMER therapy benefits include the following:

• Increased blood flow and delivery of oxygen and nutrients to all cells

2018 Update Road to Recovery from Parkinsons Disease

• Improved mitochondria function & increased production of cellular energy

• Improved cardiovascular function

• Improved cellular detoxification

• Improved athletic performance and physical fitness

• Better sleep

• Greater endurance and energy

• Better concentration and improved mental acuity

• Enhances stress reduction and relaxation

• More oxygen delivery to the brain helps improve memory & cognitive function.

BEMER isn't a "treatment" for any health condition. However, increasing delivery of oxygen and nutrients to cells and improving waste removal improves the environment within cells throughout the body and improves the body's entire ecosystem so that the body can begin to heal itself.

Some people get noticeable benefits within the first one or two sessions. However, the real benefits accrue gradually over several months of treatment. When cells have not been working well for years, supplying them with more oxygen and nutrients doesn't immediately make them work 100% efficiently.

Consider the analogy of exercise. If you haven't lifted weights or jogged for a long time, just doing one session of exercise won't make much difference in your strength or stamina. You have to work at it regularly. BEMER is much the same. Regular BEMER sessions over time dramatically accelerate the body's healing process.

The following conditions or situations are either contraindicated or you should only proceed with caution when using the BEMER:

a) People with pacemakers

b) Pregnancy

c) People on blood thinners

d) Non-titanium plates, rods, etc.

f) History of severe epilepsy

Why I Recommend the BEMER as a Preferred PEMF Device

Why do I recommend you consider the BEMER PRO as a PEMF therapy? There are many devices and options out there in the marketplace. Many of these are less expensive. The BEMER is a more sophisticated form of PEMF and, in my opinion, delivers a potentially greater benefit.

Studies clearly show that PEMF devices do offer healing benefits. This is why the "industry" has become so competitive. Studies that compare the various PEMF devices in the marketplace today place the BEMER as the most effective.

There are now a series of 20 years of R&D and numerous scientific studies published using the BEMER technology that demonstrates & documents its effectiveness. Visit www.pubmed.gov and use the search term

"BEMER therapy" to access these studies. Click HERE to access a PDF that summarizes a few of the studies that have evaluated the BEMER for various conditions.

Five international patents secure and protect BEMER's technology world-wide. PEMF is used as a delivery mechanism to send the BEMER patented energy signal into the body. BEMER PRO also has accessory devices that enable simultaneous treatment of localized areas.

I believe the most significant benefit with the BEMER is its unique sleep program. The key to attaining a return to health and wellness is to shift into a deep state of stillness while sleeping. This will enable tissues in the body to rejuvenate and regenerate. Once states of deep sleep are attained on a regular basis the body gradually returns to its natural state of balance and harmony.

Sleep cycles are regulated by brain wave frequencies. People with sleep problems have altered or dysregulated brainwave electrical activity. The BEMER Sleep Program disrupts abnormal brainwave sleep patterns and helps the electrical energy patterns of brain cells resonate or become "entrained" with normal sleep cycle brainwave frequencies. Hence, the BEMER helps reset the brain's sleep frequencies to normal/optimal frequencies required for REM sleep and deep (slow-wave) sleep cycles.

BEMER is an adaptogen.....or a normalizer. It will help to slow down frequencies that are too fast.....and it will help to speed up frequencies in people whose brainwave frequencies are too slow.

None of the BEMER competitors (that typically offer PEMF devices at a less cost) have a sleep program. BEMER Sleep mode runs for four hours each night, two hours upon going to bed and it comes on automatically again two hours before your projected wake up time. I think activating the sleep program has the potential to offer the opportunity to heal naturally from the inside out.

NASA examined all available Pulsed Electromagnetic frequency (PEMF) devices on the marketplace and concluded that the BEMER technology is the best. NASA approached BEMER and requested to be able to utilize their technology for the advanced space suit design.

On March 12, 2015, NASA and BEMER signed a cooperative agreement that governs the joint development of a prototype for a space suit to improve micro-circulation while preventing bone and muscle atrophy during space missions. It is expected that the BEMER technology & patented signal will also assist in faster recuperation after space travel.

Opportunity to Become an Independent BEMER Distributor

Acquisition of a BEMER PRO requires an initial investment of approximately $6000 which is not covered by insurance. In general, people who experience Parkinson's symptoms report to me that they experience noticeable benefits. After they start using it, they celebrate improvement in their health and wind up inviting friends and family to experience BEMER sessions themselves. Before long, people they have introduced the BEMER to decide to purchase their own units.

When you sign up to become an independent BEMER distributor (cost is only $290) you qualify to receive commissions on BEMER sales that range from 17% ($1,080) on the first four sales and 25% ($1,500) thereafter. This constitutes the company's only marketing program. They do not advertise but rather reward users for spreading the word.

I do think of the BEMER as taking on debt. It is one of the most proactive steps people can take for long-term health.

A financing option I elected to take was to apply for a CitiBank 18-month zero interest Simplicity credit card. The BEMER PRO set with taxes costs about $6,300. The payments are about $350/month. At a minimum, most people who get BEMERS end up selling enough BEMERs to offset the cost of their own personal unit.

If you are interested in discovering more about opportunities for pulsed electromagnetic field therapy whether your interest involves purchasing a BEMER PRO or exploring a rental as an option send me an email: robert@parkinsonsrecovery.com. Since I have signed up to be an Independent BEMER Distributor (having purchased a BEMER PRO myself) you can purchase BEMERS through my BEMER website. I have purchased one unit and am on the way to purchasing a second.

The company does offer a 30 day money back guarantee. However, I do not recommend that you purchase a BEMER with the intention of trying it out to see if it helps. Yes, some people report that after only a few sessions they find quick relief. However, most people who use BEMERS tell me that it takes a month or longer for them to celebrate obvious improvements in their health.

Sleep

A foundational reason why symptoms of Parkinson's emerge is a troubling imbalance between the sympathetic nervous system and the parasympathetic nervous system.

The sympathetic system is the flight-fight response. When afraid or anxious, we want to either run away from the problem or fight it directly. The parasympathetic nervous system is the nervous system that promotes rest and digestion. No one can digest their food when they are running a marathon and when standing while eating. And, no one can get to sleep if their muscles are postured to fight off a threatening and uninvited intruder into our home.

We humans survive for decades on end because both nervous systems serve vital functions. When neurological symptoms are problematic, the sympathetic fight-flight system is in control. Adrenaline and cortisol spike energy and postures us in a "get out of my way" mode of action. We are forever ready to engage with no time or opportunity to chill out, rest or digest anything including food, thoughts and feelings.

When stress is calmed and past traumas are released, you activate a dormant parasympathetic nervous system. As we all know, we can all get excited in a flash. Relaxing can easily take endless hours of meditation, soft music and pleasant company.

OK. That is the big picture. It also explains why, as neurologist Stasha Gominak MD notes, people experiencing the symptoms of Parkinson's rarely if ever drop down in the deep REM sleep that is critical for healing.

She makes the poignant argument that a person with neurological challenges will succeed in reversing their symptoms only when they succeed in getting the level of deep sleep that is critical for rejuvenating and regenerating tissues.

The problem with an overactive fight-flight sympathetic nervous system that dominates during the day is that it does not willingly give up control at night. Nope. It keeps turned on even when you sleep which is why people have difficulty sleeping. The refusal to back down is analogous to politicians who refuse to relinquish their power.

For deep healing to occur, the body has to slip down into a deep state of sleep. We become paralyzed in a good sense. A switching mechanism in the midbrain is designed to turn on (and off) temporary paralysis. With Parkinson's symptoms, the on-off switch is stuck. An overactive sympathetic nervous system keeps us tossing and turning in bed all night long.

The REM and deep sleep cycles are critical for repair and regeneration at both physical and psychic levels. People with neurological symptoms need more time in REM and deep sleep cycles because more cellular repair and rejuvenation time is needed.

Neurologist Stasha Gominak (www.drgominak.com) finds in her practice that many people have the false impression they are getting "good" sleep. She has concluded that most people with neurological challenges are not. Her view is that the root cause of neurological problems is abnormal sleep. When your sleep improves your tremor, body pain, balance problems, depression and memory loss can all improve.

Why would people believe they are getting "good" sleep every night? One possibility is that they take sleep medications. Yes, the medications do knock you out. But, they shorten and/or inhibit REM and deep sleep phases during the night. People on sleep medications tend not to get the cellular healing that emerges with states of deep sleep.

Click on the link below to hear several interviews with Dr. Gominak MD on Parkinsons Recovery Radio.

Reverse Parkinson's Symptoms with Right Sleep

Gut Brain Connection with Parkinson's

Vitamin Deficiencies
Dr. Gominak offers an eloquent explanation of the vitamin deficiencies and imbalances that

contribute to sleep problems. The key "players" in this drama of unwanted insomnia are vitamin D3, B5 (pantothenic acid), vitamin B12 (and in the end all the B vitamins). A balancing act is needed to determine the best therapeutic dosages of these key vitamins.

Vitamin D3 is the sun hormone. It is not in our food. We make D3 on our skin when we are exposed to sunshine. There is an upper limit to absorption of our skin to sun exposure of D3 which prevents the D3 blood level from rising above 80ng/ml. This level appears to be the "natural" upper limit. Supplementing vitamin D3 as a pill can easily take the D3 blood level above 80ng/ml. As it turns out, a D3 level over 80 usually makes sleep worse according to Dr. Gominak.

She offers consultations and a workbook to assist in sorting out how to proceed. It is not as simple as stuffing a bunch of vitamins down your digestive system.

She argues that a vitamin D3 deficiency causes a B12 deficiency which in turn affects sleep. A fourth of her D3 deficient patients also had an accompanying B12 deficiency. They were usually sicker as well. The B12 level for normal sleep is above 500 pg/ml.

Dr. Gominak reports on her website that:

> "Contrary to what we've all been taught, monthly B12 shots are **not** better than daily pills. The shot lasts about 3 days, and the brain needs B12 every day."

As long as you keep a watchful eye on your D3 level, she says that you are unlikely to become deficient in B12.

A vitamin D3 deficiency that is severe enough to affect sleep usually causes accompanying changes in the intestinal gut bacteria. Normal sleep requires a healthy gut biome. She suggests the following:

> "In order to bring back the "right" intestinal bacteria B-50, (a B complex that has 50 mg or 50 mcg of each of the 8 B vitamins)

should be taken for 3 months when your D blood level is over 40ng/ml. If your D level is very low and it takes a couple of months before your D level gets up above 40 ng/ml, don't start counting until your D level is 40 or above. Supplying the vitamin D and all 8 B vitamins together encourages the "right" bacteria to grow back."

The dose of vitamin D is different for each person. The key factor for good sleep is to maintain a D3 level between 60-80 ng/ml. She recommends that you check vitamin D3 blood levels several times during the initial period of adjustment to ascertain what level of D3 supplementation is needed since each person needs a different dose.

In summary, you will likely need vitamin D3 and the B vitamins supplementation to help you sleep better.

Ketone Esters

Breaking news as they say in the media: A process has been developed and refined to manufacture a concentrated source of ketones that are affordable. Several companies are now accepting orders for the new ketone ester.

Why Should Anyone with Parkinson's Symptoms Take Notice of this Development?

Ketones are a natural food for the brain. They may offer the possibility of providing temporary relief from symptoms.

How Can I be Assured this will Help with my Symptoms?

You can't! There are no systematic studies that give us any evidence one way or another. Why? The concentrated ketone ester is just now being produced commercially. The production process is lengthy and still somewhat costly although recent developments have reduced the cost significantly. It has only been made available commercially in the last few months. This really is cutting edge!

Why Hasn't a Source of Exogenous Ketone Esters Been Made Available Before?

The production cost has been prohibitive until now. What has changed? NIH researcher Richard Veech, PhD has been studying the application of ketones as a brain food for decades. He joined with University of Oxford researcher Kieran Clarke in a US Army grant to develop a food that could sustain soldiers operating in a battlefield for weeks on end. Their collaboration led to the development of methods to produce a ketone ester in the laboratory. This process is being applied now by several commercial companies.

Why the Focus on Ketones for Parkinson's?

I have been documenting natural methods that help people reverse their Parkinson's symptoms for over a decade now. Many wonderful therapies and treatments have been identified and documented, all of which help most people to one degree or another.

What about those of you who have been taking medications for a number of years with good results, but your "time on" periods are shorter and shorter? You may be in a situation where your doctor is no longer willing to prescribe a higher dose. If so, what are your options now?

Surgery is an option that helps some people but not others. I realize many of you do not want to pursue that option. The ketone ester may be an option that will extend the viability of taking medicines to suppress the symptoms.

Keep in mind that the ketone ester, like medicines, is also a temporary "fix." Depending on the person and the dose, relief is several hours or hopefully longer. The good news is that you will know if the ester helps within 20-30 minutes after taking it (or even sooner).

It is my hope – and it is just that – that the new concentrated external source of ketones may provide the boost needed to get your life back if you are in just this situation. If you decide to give it a try – please give me feedback.

The Big Picture for Ketones as I See It

Research shows that the people who live longer, healthier lives eat less. Why is this?

Partly, they fast at least 12-18 hours a day. Fasting encourages the liver to make ketones (approximately 150 grams a day). Ketones are the "natural" brain food. They require less energy for the body to process.

The brain also functions on glucose. The body converts carbs and proteins into sugar/glucose which the brain uses to function.

The video posted at the top of the the www.ketoneaid.com website listed below provides a brief overview of the history behind producing a commercially viable ester. There are quite a few testimonials from athletes who experience a noticeable boost in their performance that are also posted down this website. Because the ester is new there is no research evidence to support its application for neurological conditions so the company wisely chose to make no claims about its potential for any illness including Parkinson's.

www.ketoneaid.com

There is a marvelous analogy to building a fire with regard to what happens when we eat carbs, proteins and fat. We all know that you can build and maintain a campfire with kindling, wood and/or charcoal. Kindling burns fast. It is similar to the fast acting brain fuel when we eat carbs. Protein is more like burning wood. The food burns longer as does the effect of eating protein to produce brain fuel. Finally, fat is like burning charcoal which burns a long time. Eating fat facilitates the production of ketones. As a natural brain food, ketones are by for the longest lasting fuel for the brain.

There is an on/off switch at play here. Either the body is using sugar to fuel the brain (from the carbs and proteins) or it is extracting ketones from stores of fat. When sugar is the primary fuel, the body is working on overtime and not getting paid for it! When ketones are the primary fuel, demands on the body are significantly less (which is why life is extended). In short -

- Ketones are easy for the body to process
- Sugar is not.

This is why eating sweets (that have raw sugar) is not a smart idea for persons with neurological challenges. Yes, it creates glucose which is food for your brain. But, the fuel it offers to the brain to sustain brain function is short lasting. This is why ingesting sugar can cause brain fog and why ketones provide a sharp edge to mental functioning.

How Ketones Can Be Produced in the Body
There are various methods that can be used in combination to facilitate the production of ketones in your body. I recommend that you consider adopting a combination of these methods rather than depending on taking the new ketone ester alone. Given the expense of the ketone ester, it is not a day in and day out option for most people.

The options are described below and include the ketone ester, fasting, a high fat diet and a ketone salt. Bill Curtis explains how he uses a combination of approaches during my interview with him on Parkinsons Recovery Radio.

2018 Update Road to Recovery from Parkinsons Disease

During the interview Bill talks about his efforts to understand how ketones help with his Parkinson's symptoms. He developed Parkinson's symptoms at the age of 45 in the year 2000 and has been instrumental in collaborating with NIH researcher Richard Veech in Washington DC over the last several years.

What follows are the questions I asked Bill during the interview on Parkinsons Recovery Radio.

Interview with Bill Curtis on Parkinsons Recovery Radio

- *How did Parkinson's affect your life?*
- *What led you to experiment with ketosis?*
- *After the ketogenic exercise, what did you do to find out more about how ketosis could help your Parkinson's symptoms?*
- *What is the purpose of fasting?*
- *What is the purpose of the morning fat and coffee mixture?*
- *What happens when you eat too much carbohydrate?*

- *What happens when you eat too much protein?*
- *Can exercise take you out of ketosis?*
- *Can stress take you out of ketosis?*
- *What supplements do you take to support ketosis?*
- *What do you think is causing the improvement in symptoms?*
- *Have you been able to cut back on the Parkinson's medications?*
- *What do you think is going on as far as the disease progression you personally are experiencing?*
- *Where do you think the use of ketosis in Parkinson's is going?*

Fasting

Fasting is one sure bet to facilitate the production of ketones in your body. Many people shun the idea of fasting because they think it means not eating for days on end. Fasting can be effortless if practiced on a daily basis.

The easy way to fast is simply to eat the last meal of the day in the early evening. Then, do not eat anything for 12-14 hours until the following morning. Make this a daily habit. There is no need to set aside 4 days or longer to stop eating food.

High Fat Diet

Eating a fat rich diet with few carbs and little protein – known as a ketogenic diet – also facilitates the production of ketones. Ketones are produced in the liver from fat.

Doctors will sometimes recommend a high fat diet for persons with epileptic fits because the natural production of ketones as fuel for the brain has been found to reduce the frequency and severity of seizures.

The ketogenic diet is a high-fat, limited protein and carbohydrate diet that encourages the body to burn fat. When we eat carbohydrates, they convert to glucose which becomes fuel to sustain brain functions. When there is little to no carbohydrates that are ingested, your liver converts fat into and ketone bodies. The ketones become natural food for your brain rather than using glucose as an energy source.

Drinking a cocktail in the morning consisting of a drink composed of coffee, butter, whipped cream and coconut oil (and/or MCT oil) is used by some persons with Parkinson's who pursue a ketone diet. The body uses these fats to product ketones.

Naturopath Bruce Fife ND has written a series of marvelous books on how to cook with coconut oils and coconut sugars. If you are interested in adding a little healthy fat to your diet, listen to my interview with Dr. Fife on Parkinson's Recovery Radio. You will be sold on coconut as a food after listening to the replay of this interview. You will also be inspired to make healthy desserts.

Healing Potential of Coconut Oil and Coconut Sugar

Ketone Salts

Still another source of ketones can be acquired from ingesting ketone salts. Taking salts does not give you a huge boast in ketones - certainly nothing close to taking the ketone ester or even fasting. Some people take salts as one among other ways to facilitate the production of ketones in their bodies. Ketone salts are certainly less expensive than the ester, but limited in the quantity of ketones that can be generated.

There are many ketone salt options that are available from various sources. The preferred options are certainly not the cheapest. Frank Llosa, the CEO of Ketoneaid.com, recommends a MAX ketone salt offered by Pruvitnow. Their ketone salt products can be purchased from the following website:
https://ourkeytolife.shopketo.com

Ketone Ester

Presently the cost of purchasing the ketone ester remains somewhat pricey but certainly less than the cost of many other alternatives (such as some medicines and surgeries). One gram costs on average $1 now. The costs of production are being reduced as the production process is refined. Producing the ester in larger quantities will also bring the cost down eventually.

A single ketone ester treatment for me – I weigh 155 pounds, is approximately 35 grams or $35. People who weigh more have to take more of the external ketone. This may sound pricey – but it is a bargain compared to a year ago. Some people can take half this much and get just as much relief from their symptoms.

The cost of producing a single gram of the ketone ester a year ago was $1,000. Obviously, great strides have been made with developing a cost effective production process.

Still, it does not seem reasonable for most people to take the ketone ester as a sole source of symptom relief every day. With a little experimentation, it may be you supplement the ester with the other methods that produce ketones. This is precisely what Bill Curtis does.

2018 Update Road to Recovery from Parkinsons Disease

The ester will give a quick boost (usually of mental clarity and energy) but it is, relatively speaking, an expensive boost. Bill Curtis reports that he uses the ester in selective circumstances (such as when he is stressed) as a way of counteracting the lactic acid produced by exercise or when he has a particularly challenging task to perform whether at work or at play.

How to Purchase the Ketone Ester

If you wait to order there is a strong likelihood orders will be closed temporarily. As noted, this is a new production process. It takes time to produce the ketone ester in the lab. Demand for the ester is off the charts – particularly from competitive athletes who are willing to spend any amount of money to gain a competitive advantage. (Please note: Professional sports teams are waiting in line to purchase the ester when it becomes available).

Frank Llosa, the CEO of www.ketoneaid.com has currently opened up orders of the ketone ester. Cost for a trainer bottle is $300. Enter the coupon code **Zero** on the shopping cart to qualify for free shipping. If you put off ordering, you may well discover the opportunity to order will be shut down until more of the ester becomes available. Of course, you can always wait for the opportunity to order again, but you may have to wait months as has been the experience recently. The website where you can submit an order is:

www.ketoneaid.com/buy

I suspect some of you are probably thinking – right. The company is putting a fake deadline on purchasing which, from a marketing point of view, always triggers more sales. I want you all to know that this is no marketing ploy or manipulation. If you wait to try the ketone ester, supply will very likely be exhausted. Because the commercial availability of the ketone ester is so new, supplies are limited. In short, if this option for recovery calls out to you, I suggest you purchase the ester and give it a trial run now.

To summarize - I think Bill Curtis has an ideal approach. Do some experimentation and use a combination of the various options that can facilitate the production of ketones in your body including the ketone ester, high fat diet (possibly), fasting and ketone salts. Develop your own approach using a combination of some or all of the above options.

The liver manufactures about on average 150 grams of ketones a day, so you can produce ketones using any of the variety of methods listed above. Why not set the intention to feed your brain with the natural food it needs to function at its highest capacity of clarity and focus rather than relying on glucose as its primary fuel source? Does that seem to be a smart way to feed your brain?

CBD Oil

Mounting anecdotal evidence indicates that CBD has the potential to offer temporary relief from the symptoms associated of Parkinson's disease. To view the wide range of experiences reported by persons diagnosed with Parkinson's disease, visit www.youtube.com and search on the terms "CBD Parkinson's" or some variant thereof.

What is CBD?

CBD stands for "cannabidiol oil." It can be extracted from either the hemp plant or the marijuana plant. Taking CBD oil gives users the medical benefits of medical marijuana without the high that is associated with THC found in Marijuana. CBD derived from the hemp plant itself has no psychedelic properties and is considered safe for consumption.

Impact of CBD on Parkinson's Symptoms is Temporary

Use of CBD offers symptomatic suppression of Parkinson's symptoms much like medications and supplements. If your symptoms are to the point of interfering with an ability to live a full and vibrant life, then you clearly do not have the energy, focus or motivation to formulate a realistic healing program to reverse the symptoms. Obviously, any initiative that is needed to kick start a recovery program is impossible to launch when you are feeling lousy. Use of CBD may just provide the kick start you need to launch a successful journey down the road to recovery.

Research on CBD and Parkinson's

Research (although limited) suggests that use of CBD may well offer the opportunity to get temporary relief from symptoms. This is a valuable benefit in itself. When energy, focus and motivation return, the business of taking the actions necessary to heal from the inside out can begin at long last.

Cannabidiol (CBD) is one of at least 85 active cannabinoids. Scientific studies are reporting a wide variety of positive health benefits. CBD has been found to be helpful to the endocannabinoid system. Many scientific discoveries link poor health to endocannabinoid deficiencies.

Studies have found positive effects for the use of CBD on anxiety, stress and PTSD. You can find these studies listed at pubmed.com (the US government's index of scientific studies). Search the terms "CBD anxiety."

Below are listed abstracts from the few recent studies that have examined the effects of CBD on subjects who currently experience Parkinson's symptoms.

Effects of cannabidiol in the treatment of patients with Parkinson's disease: an exploratory double-blind trial.

J Psychopharmacol. 2014 Nov;28(11):1088-98. doi: 10.1177/0269881114550355. Epub 2014 Sep 18.

Chagas MH, Zuardi AW, Tumas V, Pena-Pereira MA, Sobreira ET, Bergamaschi MM, dos Santos AC, Teixeira AL, Hallak JE, Crippa JA.

2018 Update Road to Recovery from Parkinsons Disease

Twenty one (21) subjects were assigned to three groups of seven subjects each who were treated with placebo, cannabidiol (CBD) 75 mg/day or CBD 300 mg/day. One week before the trial and in the last week of treatment subjects were evaluated with respect to motor and general symptoms score (UPDRS) and well-being and quality of life (PDQ-39).

Despite the very small sample size, groups treated with placebo and **CBD 300 mg/day** had significantly different mean total scores in the PDQ-39 (p = 0.05). Significance is very much a factor of sample size, so this result is striking in itself. Findings suggest a possible effect of CBD in improving quality of life measures in PD patients with no psychiatric comorbidities.

Cannabidiol can improve complex sleep-related behaviours associated with rapid eye movement sleep behaviour disorder in Parkinson's disease patients: a case series.

J Clin Pharm Ther. 2014 Oct;39(5):564-6. doi: 10.1111/jcpt.12179. Epub 2014 May 21

2018 Update Road to Recovery from Parkinsons Disease

Chagas MH, Eckeli AL, Zuardi AW, Pena-Pereira MA, Sobreira-Neto MA, Sobreira ET, Camilo MR, Bergamaschi MM, Schenck CH, Hallak JE, Tumas V, Crippa JA.

The administration of cannabidiol (CBD) was found to control sleep disorders in patients who currently experience the symptoms of Parkinson's disease as reported in the *Journal of Clinical Pharmacy and Therapeutics*. An international team of researchers from the University of Sao Paulo in Brazil and the University of Minnesota Medical School USA evaluated the ingestion of CBD by four Parkinson's disease patients with REM sleep behavior disorder (RBD). This condition is characterized by nightmares and active behavior during dreaming.

Cannabidiol treatment reduced symptoms in each of the four subjects. Symptoms returned with the same frequency and intensity following subjects' discontinuation of the cannabinoid.

IS CBD Oil Legal in All States?

The answer is – at long last – yes. CBD can legality be sold and shipped to residents of all US states as well as many European countries. It is not legal in all countries.

What are Potential Side Effects from Taking CBD Oil?

There are a few minor negative side effects that result for some users of CBD oil including low blood pressure, light headedness, fatigue, dry mouth, and slowed motor functions. In the majority of studies, these side effects have been reported to be mild.

Bottom Line

The CBD therapy seems to be a good one to consider, especially if you are having significant challenges functioning independently on a day to day basis. As with any natural treatment option, be sure to check with your doctor to insure that use of CBD will not interfere with any treatments your doctor has prescribed for you.

Recommendation for a High Quality, Low Cost Source of 1500 mg CBD Oil

Parkinsons Recovery has been at the forefront of documenting new and promising therapies that offer the potential to address symptoms of Parkinson's disease. Three years ago I documented on Parkinsons Recovery radio and on the blog the potential usefulness of CBD oils as a therapy for Parkinson's. The CBD company I hosted on the radio show in 2016 offered high quality CBD with a 300 mg concentration. The price was high. Since the interview, they have struggled to remain in business.

With the passage of a few years, new companies have emerged that offer CBD with higher potency concentrations. This clearly is an exploding market. I have been hesitant to recommend any source of CBD oils until recently when a member of my audience suggested I investigate a CBD company called CTFO. My due diligence led me to conclude that this company offers customers exactly what we all want: high quality CBD, high concentration and the lowest wholesale cost of any CBD company in the marketplace. I want you to know about this company so you can do your own due diligence.

The following sections detail information about the CBD oils offered by a CTFO. Now, if you currently purchase CBD oil from a reliable source and are pleased with the results - you might as well skip the following section.

If however, your answer to the following questions is yes, you may very well find the information about this specific product to be very worthwhile.

- *Have you been using CBD oils to address Parkinson's symptoms?*
- *Have you been on the lookout for a high quality source at an affordable cost? The oils can get pricey if you use them on a regular basis.*

CTFO sells high quality CBD oils at an affordable and very competitive pricing. They also sell a CBD oil with a high concentration (1500 mg) which you do not see with the product offerings of most companies. More commonly, companies offer the oils at lower concentrations from 25 mg to 300 mg.

Have you wanted to try taking CBD oil to suppress your symptoms but have not done so yet? Perhaps you did not take action because it involved spending money on something you did not know would help.

This particular company (CTFO) offers a 60 day money back guarantee. This means that you can purchase the high concentration **1500 mg CBD** oil, take the entire bottle (which incidentally will last you about a month) and receive a full refund by simply returning the empty bottle (within 60 days after purchase) if taking the 1500 mg CBD oil does not offer the relief you were expecting. The company extends this generous offer because most people discover the oils are helpful.

There will only be a little expense involved with return shipping and handling. All in all, you get to try out this as a potential therapy without worrying you will be spending money on a therapy that does not help. As I see matters, this company is offering everyone a virtually cost free opportunity to try it out. Why not order some CBD oil and see for yourself whether it helps. This quickly resolves all speculation!

Application and Use of CBD Oils for Parkinson's is a New Development

Important Qualification: You may not be able to purchase the CTFO oils depending on where you live. The CTFO oils are currently shipped only to addresses in the United States, Great Britain, Scotland, Wales, Northern Ireland, Ireland and Sweden. Shipments to Canada will be available soon.

I signed up to be an affiliate of the company for free. You can do the same. When I refer others to try the CTFO CBD products, I have the opportunity to cover the cost of my own CBD oils. Or, you can always simply be a customer and not bother registering as an associate with the company.

What is the difference between CBD Herbal Drops and Isolate CBD Drops?
Neither product causes any hallucinations or highs. The Herbal CBD does contain an extremely

small amount of TCP (the chemical that does cause a "high.") There is a very small possibility that testing for drug use could possibly flag a problem. Isolate CBD drops can be taken without worrying that any residue of TCP will be picked up in a blood test.

If you have an occupation that requires routine drug testing, you will need to order and take the Isolate. All other persons should order and take the herbal drops which have greater potency and effectiveness. Again, you do not have to worry about getting "high" taking either product.

Below is a link to the website CTFO set up for Parkinsons Recovery with the information on the various CBD oil products they offer. From this website you too can register for free to become an associate of the company or simply purchase the oils as a customer.

I will be using the revenues generated from my affiliation with the company to cover the cost of the oils I purchase and to subsidize the many free services I offer through Parkinsons Recovery.

http://parkinsonsrecovery.myctfocbd.com/

Macrobiotics

Over the past decade I have hosted a number of guests who have suggested one diet plan or another that might potentially help address symptoms of Parkinson's disease. Each guest is an expert in their own right with solid evidence to support their recommendations. Still, which of the various recommendations should be put into action? I have been puzzled with an answer I could offer with some degree of confidence. Every interview is so convincing!

Until that is when I hosted an interview with Warren Kramer on Parkinsons Recovery Radio (macrobioticsnewengland.com). Click the link below to hear the full interview.

The Macrobiotic Approach

Warren is a mentor and teacher to many persons over the past 30 years who have experienced Parkinson's symptoms. His suggestions and recommendations are based on extensive experience working closely with persons who experience neurological symptoms (as well as other conditions as well). His recommendations are all about how we can heal by avoiding the wrong food and eating the right foods. An accounting of his recommendations and insights follow.

When and How Should You Eat?

Most people believe that the only important decision involves what you eat. What about when and how? Warren reports that even if you make no changes to your dietary intake, you can celebrate improvement in your health and wellbeing by establishing a routine of when and how you eat.

> *When should you eat?* Eat at regular times during the day. For example, eat your first meal between 7:00 am and 8:00 am, lunch between 12:00 and 1:00 pm and dinner between 6:00 and 7:00. Do not eat meals late at night and certainly not after dinner.
>
> *How should you eat?* Simple. Sit down when you eat. Do not eat standing up and on the run.

What Can Always Help Me Feel Better?

Stop eating foods that are causing trouble for you. This may be foods that you are allergic to. Warren reports that over the course of his 30 years of helping people, everyone feels better when they stop eating sugar. Everyone. No exceptions.

Warren describes symptoms of Parkinson's disease as fitting into two general categories: (1) quick movements (such as persons with tremors) and (2) Slow movements (such as those with movement challenges). He then suggests specific foods to avoid depending on which category describes you.

Foods to avoid if you have quick movements.

Warren recommends that persons who fall into this category (otherwise described as yang energy), should stop eating animal foods and baked goods that contain flour. When they do, tremors should quiet down.

Foods to avoid if you have slow movements

Warren recommends that persons who fall into this category (otherwise described as yin energy) should avoid eating sweets, white flour, bananas, fruit juice and of course alcohol (which contains a lot of sugar).

Treatment for Tremors

Warren recommends a home remedy that he finds has been successful for calming tremors. The preparation includes three ingredients and takes 10 minutes to prepare. The preparation should be made each day so that it is fresh and contains high energy.

Ingredients for the Tremor Treatment
½ Umeboshi Plum
Kuzu - 1 teaspoon
Tamari sauce (few drops depending on taste)

Recipe
Add one teaspoon of Kuzu to one cup of water. Bring to a boil. Add ½ of a Umeboshi Plum. Put several drops of Tamari source. Drink hot.

This daily preparation strengthens the vibrancy of the intestines and helps control tremors. Warren recommends that you prepare and drink the tremor preparation every day for 2-3 weeks, then continue with drinking the preparation every other day.

The ingredient of Kuzu may be vaguely familiar to those of you who live in the southern United States. He reports this is the same family as Kudzu vine that you see growing all over the place! When kuzu is purchased, it takes the form of a white powder.

Warren recommended that a high quality, organic source of the Umeboshi plum and kuzu is from the following company: www.healthgoods.com. I purchased both products from this website. Total cost including shipping was $45.

Natural Treatment to Facilitate More Movement in the Body

Grate a ginger root. Separate out the pulp from the juice. Dip a towel into a bowl containing water and the juice you have extracted from the ginger root. Ring out the excess water from the towel. Then, rub towel up and down the spine. It helps to have someone else help you with this – though you can also do this yourself with a big enough towel. Do this every day. It helps improve circulation and facilitates more movement in the body.

Having Trouble Changing your Diet?

You are certainly not alone. Everyone has problems breaking bad habits. Hey. We all have bad habits we need to change. Here is the good news. **Food craves food.** If a lifetime habit of yours has been to eat hamburgers at fast food chains, your body will continue to crave eating hamburgers at fast food chains even when you know this habit is bad for you.

When you start eating nutritious foods, your body will gradually crave more of the nutritious foods. When you shift a habit, it will be a challenge in the early days. But, hang in there! Eventually your body will rebel at the prospect of eating fast food because it now craves fresh, organic, live food.

Foods Recommended for Persons with Parkinson's Symptoms

A fascinating recommendation Warren offers is to avoid eating cold salads. He recommends eating warm, cooked veggies that can be blanched, steamed or sautéed. Included on the recommended list are slow cooked foods like squash, sweet potatoes, carrots, burdock root, carrots, lentils and beans with a little sea salt. Homemade miso soup is also one of the dishes on the top of his recommended list for Parkinson's.

Food to Heal Distressed Kidneys

It is well documented that toxins play a central role with Parkinson's. A key reason for the toxic overload is a person's kidneys are compromised and are unable to discharge the toxins. What food helps bring kidneys back into full functionality?

Beans! He points out the obvious. The shape of many beans is precisely the same shape as kidney. Eat kidney beans to strengthen the capacity of your kidney to eliminate toxins.

Amino Acid Therapy

Marty Hinz MD is the pioneer in advocating amino acid therapy for addressing symptoms of Parkinson's disease. His research into amino acid therapy spans 21 years. Click below to access the replay of my interview with Dr. Hinz MD and his associate Ross Stuart PhD.

All About Amino Acid Therapy With Dr. Marty Hinz MD and Ross Stuart PhD

Amino acid therapy focuses on repairing damaged cells in the substantia nigra (located in the midbrain) that produce dopamine. This compromises the efficient transmission of messages across the neural networks that, in turn, affect fine motor control.

The most effective treatment is l-dopa, one among many amino acids that converts into dopamine. The issue with L-dopa is that it has troubling side effects such as nausea which makes it intolerable to take without additional support to control its nasty side effects.

The most commonly prescribed L-dopa medication is Sinemet which is a prescribed medicine taken by many people that contains not only l-dopa but also carbidopa. Carbidopa is included in Sinemet to control the side effects of L-dopa. It has no independent therapeutic value other than helping to control the side effects of L-dopa.

Dr. Hinz explains that carbidopa causes depletions of essential vitamins and nutrients which over the long run become unmanageable. His approach is to manage the side effects of l-dopa by balancing and adjusting the many other amino acids instead of adding carbidopa.

Issues with Carbidopa

What are the issues with carbidopa? It binds to vitamin B6 and eventually takes B6 out of the body. Vitamin B6 deficiency is problematic for a number of reasons. It is associated with an increased death rate due to heart attacks and lung problems. Even more problematic is the fact that the enzyme that converts l-dopa to dopamine is – you guessed it – vitamin B6.

We are not even done yet! One of the body's natural defenses against neuro-toxins is glutathione. Many people with Parkinson's symptoms have a serious deficiency of glutathione. The substantia nigra has been shown to have a low level of glutathione which makes it particularly susceptible to damage from neuro-toxins.

Dr. Hinz explains that the critical vitamin needed for the body to produce glutathione is – here it is again - vitamin B6. When B6 is depleted, the body's defense against neuro-toxins is disabled.

In summary, L-dopa is an effective therapy, but people cannot take it independently because of the troubling side effects. Carbidopa has been added to l-dopa in prescription medications to quiet the side effects, but this in turn depletes a foundational vitamin – B6 - necessary to dopamine production. Dr. Hinz explains that many Parkinson's patients are deficient in vitamin B6, so their bodies are not making the dopamine they need.

Dr Hinz believes that amino acid therapy is preferable to adding carbidopa to L-dopa. He makes delicate adjustments to various amino acids to get l-dopa working without its troubling side effects. Eventually, he reports that his patients get better. Patients do require many weeks of ongoing adjustments to get a person "straightened out."

Why Not Just Take More B6?

This is probably your question too. I asked Dr. Hinz why a deficiency in B6 could not be simply solved by taking a B6 supplement. He explained this is never the solution. When a person takes enough B6 to neutralize the carbidopa, they will be "clobbered" with headaches.

Mechanics of Amino Acid Therapy

L-dopa collapses as many as 29 other systems in the body. Controlling its side effects involves a delicate balancing act of many amino acids which must be closely monitored by a doctor who follows Dr. Hinz's protocols. A systematic program of adjustments is prescribed on a weekly basis. Recommendations are now down to a "science". When a patient experiences "X", the doctor will recommend "Y". Both Dr. Hinz and Dr. Stuart emphasize that the adjustments are not guesswork.

Every patient has to be managed on a week to week basis. Each person's requirements will be different. Amino acid therapy is not something you can figure out without a doctor's ongoing consultations.

Ross Stuart PhD reports that the amino acid program is not for the "faint of heart". He requires his patients to commit "up front" to 24 weeks of week to week consultations using teleseminar conferencing. No visits to a doctor's office are required. Blood tests are not usually used, but urine tests may be requested after the initial period of 5-6 weeks or so. Cost of each consultation is $125. Expenditures for the amino acids is an additional expense to be incurred. An upfront financial commitment is required of each patient that covers a full 24 weeks of treatment.

Additional information is available on two websites: Ross Stuart's website: www.bbwca.com

and Dr. Hinz's website (which contains information on his amino acid research publications) www.parkinsonsclinics.com

They see patients from all over the world and caution it is not an "easy" program or simple "fix." Adjustment of amino acids has to be precise to address a person's individual needs and requirements.

Ross Stuart emphasizes you have to be persistent. It will take a while to help a patient get adjusted given their unique chemistry. You very well may get sick a few times. "There is always darkness before the dawn." Many of their patients have digestive disorders which have to be addressed. Dr. Stuart cautions not to expect much improvement over the initial 6-8 weeks, but after that initial period, most patients begin to feel better.

Who is Most Helped by Amino Acid Therapy?
Both Dr. Hinz and Dr. Stuart emphasize that their amino acid therapy is most successful for persons who are in the early rather than later stages. Their best successes are with persons who have

just been diagnosed. They do not see much improvement if a person's symptoms have significantly progressed. The longer a person has been taking Sinemet they longer it takes to regulate and the more l-dopa will be required. In some cases patients with advanced symptoms may require a higher dose of l-dopa that is actually contained in Sinemet.

To this end the amino acid clinics initially screen patients to assess whether the therapy can be beneficial. They only accept people as new patients who have a good chance of success. They also limit how many new patients they accept into their program.

Amino acid therapy helps to manage symptoms. It does not address the underlying factors that cause them. If a patient stops taking the amino acids, their symptoms will resurface.

There is a substantial difference between what Dr. Hinz recommends to his patients and what most neurologists recommend to their patients. For a patient with a recent diagnosis, he will start them taking L-dopa immediately and follow his amino acid protocol. Most neurologists recommend to hold off taking Sinemet (which contains l-dopa) if they have a recent diagnosis.

You can contact Dr. Hinz's office by calling 0877-626-2220 or visiting his website:

www.neurosupport.com

Printed in Great Britain
by Amazon